CHEMOTHERAPY
Gives New Meaning To A Bad Hair Day

A Healing Book

EILEEN MARIN
Illustrations by Michael Weber

First edition published 1995

Marin, Eileen

       Chemotherapy Gives New Meaning To A Bad Hair Day
       1. Cancer - Chemotherapy 2. Health 3. Healing
       4. Inspiration I. Title II. Author

Library of Congress Catalog Card Number 95-78619
ISBN 1-885676-085

DEDICATION

This book is dedicated to the friends I knew,
the friends I know and the friends I have yet
to meet who share the cancer experience ...

One Day At A Time.

A NOTE

A percentage of each book sold will be donated to a
number of non-profit cancer related organizations and
foundations.

If you purchased this book through a hospital,
or doctor affiliated with a hospital, the percentage will
be donated to that specific hospital's cancer center.

Recipe For Cancer Survivors

2   Cups Laughter
1/4   Cup Tears
1   Day At A Time
2+   Supportive Friends
1   Heart Of Love

Mix laughter with tears. Sprinkle liberally with supportive friends who listen. Do this one day at a time with love.

Foreword

People with cancer often feel frightened and alone. But, if the cancer patient masters a positive outlook, liberally laced with humor, other people will want to be around them. From a clinical standpoint, laughter increases endorphins, which are natural chemicals in the body that diminish pain and promote an overall sensation of well-being. They may even prolong survival by enhancing the immune system.

Unfortunately, you can't always control whether or not you get cancer. However, you can choose how you react to your disease.

Tears, like a cleansing rain, are not only inevitable but beneficial. Anger, too, is a healthy short-term reaction. But humor and acceptance make friendly companions on the road ahead. You get to choose.

Remember, the greatest enemy of humor is fear. Laughter drives away demons and other negative spirits that thrive in darkness. And, if you laugh enough, you don't have to do sit ups!

Janet Hale, M.D.
Medical City, Dallas

CHEMOTHERAPY GIVES NEW MEANING TO A BAD HAIR DAY

My Story

My first experience with *Eileen, I'm sorry but...* was in January 1992. My life was good. I was 44, eating healthy, exercising, and meditating. I was also self-employed with no health insurance. I accepted my diagnosis, had two surgeries, faced radiation therapy and continued on with my life. The most important part of each day was a dose of humor; mine and that of some television shows or tapes that always struck me funny. I bought books for a friend diagnosed with breast cancer the year before. I borrowed them, bought more and gathered all the information I could on my disease, the treatments and the alternatives.

The second time I heard *Eileen, I'm sorry but ...* was in February 1992. I was face-to-face with additional surgeries and an empty bank book. I was not too happy when I realized my surgeries and subsequent treatments were going to be at the county hospital. My positive attitude was put to the test. My meditation and visualization techniques helped me get through the ten-hour days waiting for doctors and treatments. As they say in kindergarten, I used my time wisely. I talked to other patients about how I was coping and shared my books, tapes and thoughts. My sense of humor returned and my mantra was *if it's Tuesday, I must be in surgery.* I looked at the whole year of surgeries, chemotherapy and radiation treatments as a once in a lifetime experience. And, was overjoyed at the end of the year when it was completed. I started a new job in the middle of my treatments. I continued taking my vitamins and using my juicer as I had during the year of surgeries and treatments. My only reminders of the cancer were periodic doctor visits. The third time I heard the words *Eileen, I'm sorry but ...* was in July 1994. I did not accept this diagnosis very gracefully. I was in shock; how could this happen again? I was taking such good care of myself.

I was filled with a great deal of anger and confusion but knew enough to ask for help. Working with an oncology social worker at the hospital and attending support group meetings helped me put this third diagnosis into prospective. Again, my saving grace was my sense of humor; *this time I had health insurance and sick leave.*

Although it may sound strange to some, I look at my diagnoses as a blessing. It is only through the cancer experiences that I am able to know and be my true self — and, most of all, take the risks necessary to live life to its fullest *one day at a time.*

It is with love and appreciation that I thank my four skilled surgeons:

Dr. Janet Hale [Medical City/Dallas],
Dr. Marilyn Leach [Parkland Hospital/Dallas],
Dr. Frances Crites and Dr. Marcus Downs
[Presbyterian Hospital/Dallas].

I also want to thank:

- My friends who racked up frequent driver miles taking me back and forth to emergency rooms and *designated driver* procedures.

- Donna, who provided the reason to put the cartoons and thoughts on paper.

- Judi, sister by birth and friend by choice, who actively supported me and cried in silence. My mother Ellie who supported the telephone company and the card store. My son Jaye, for just being, and keeping daily life and routines from changing very much in the light of three cancer diagnoses and treatments.

- Lisa (LB) Bear who went through as many surgeries, hospital stays and treatments as I did. And, listened to me with unconditional love and understanding at all hours of the day and night.

Most important, I am grateful to the divine presence in my life that has guided my thoughts and actions, has placed special people on my path, and made this book a reality.

Support yourself and cancer research...let's find a cure that doesn't include throwing up!

Introduction

There are so many excellent books on meditation and visualization; questions and answers on cancer and its treatments and the importance of humor when coping with illness or wellness. Knowledge is power ... arm yourself with all the resources that are available. Some prescriptions do not have to be filled at a pharmacy. Some can be filled at the book store or library. You don't have to be an author or an artist to use their techniques of writing, sketching or scribbling to express feelings. Let the sayings and illustrations in this book trigger your feelings and experiences. Use the blank pages to write a word, a sentence or a paragraph. Draw an elaborate picture, sketch, doodle or scribble to let out the angry, sad, happy and glad feelings of each day.

Life is not a dress rehearsal.
Make each day count.

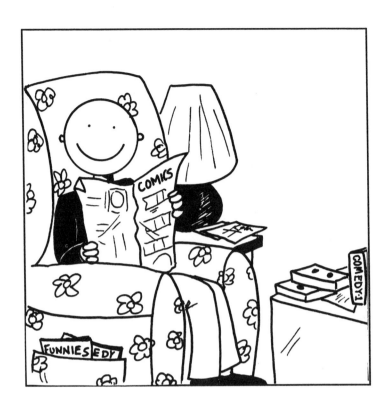

Laughter is the best medicine.
It's free and doesn't have to be filed
with insurance.

Oh no, not another test that requires a designated driver.

CHEMOTHERAPY GIVES NEW MEANING TO A BAD HAIR DAY

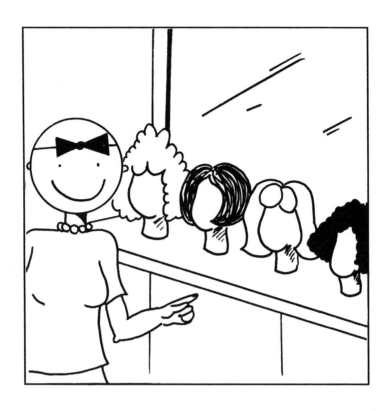

Decisions - decisions - decisions.
Think I'll be a red head today.

Be real. Be honest. Talk about it.
Ask for what you need.

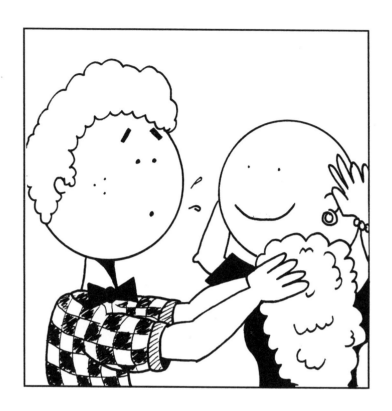

And then he ran his fingers through
my hair. Surprise!

I think of prayers as the cement that holds medical treatments in place.

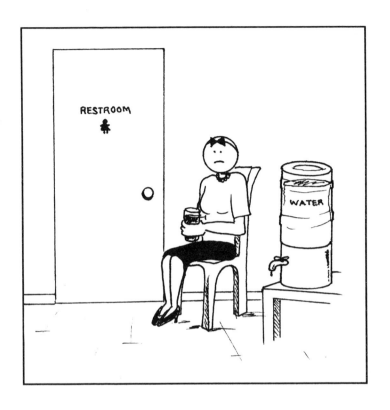

You want me to drink how many
gallons and not use what?

13

*Cancer is the ultimate wake up call.
What are the major priorities
in your life?*

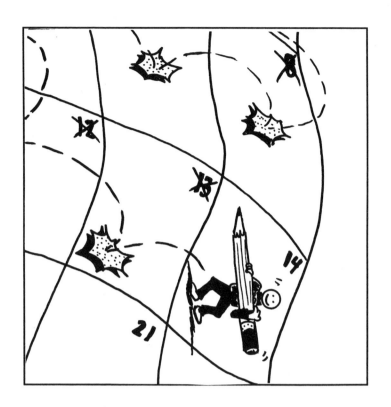

One day at a time is manageable.

*Looking back will I say I should have
spent more time at work?*

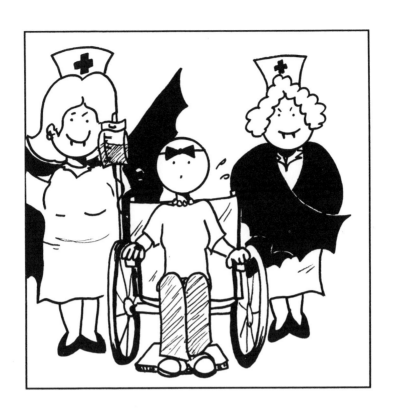

Some nurses are vampire clones.

Reach out and help someone.
Share your hope — not horror stories.

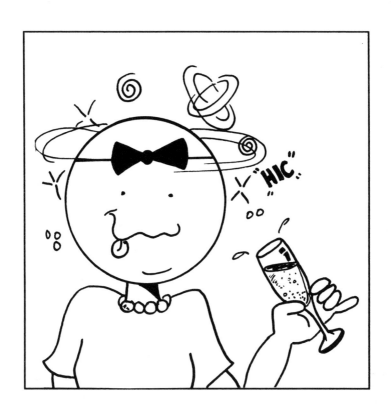

I remember when port referred
to a type of wine.

What is important anyway?

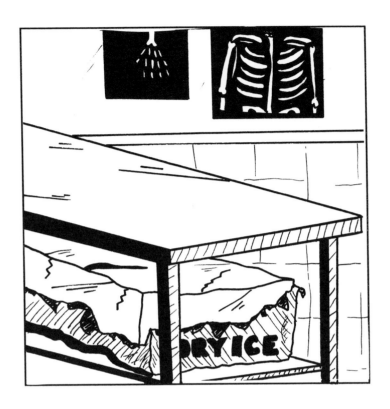

How do they regulate the temperature
of the X-ray table to consistently
read frigid?

*It's time to stop thinking about that trip
or class and take an action.*

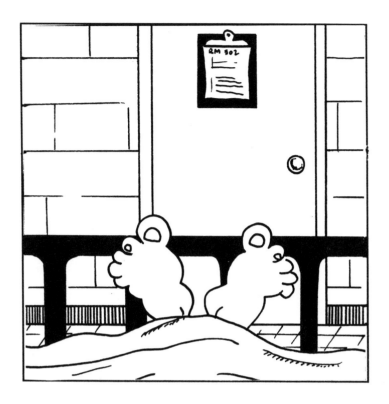

The kids prefer talking about cancer of the toe rather than embarassing breast, colon and prostate cancer.

Caring friends will remain close and supportive. Cancer is a weeding out process.

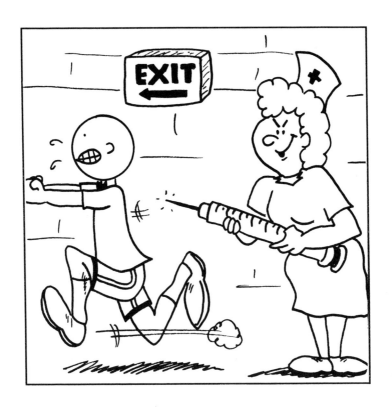

Fear is toxic.
It affects the mind and the body.

Don't sweat the small stuff.
It's all small stuff.

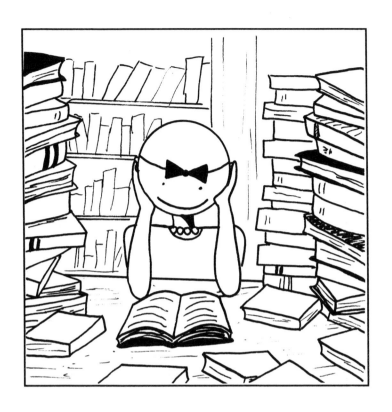

Knowledge is power.
Arm yourself with information.

They went to school for years to tell me how to do what?

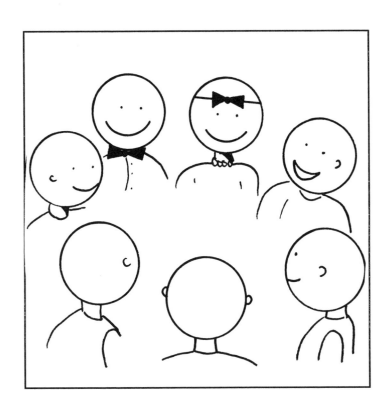

Some of my best friends have
been bald.

You mean it's just a run of the mill ordinary headache?

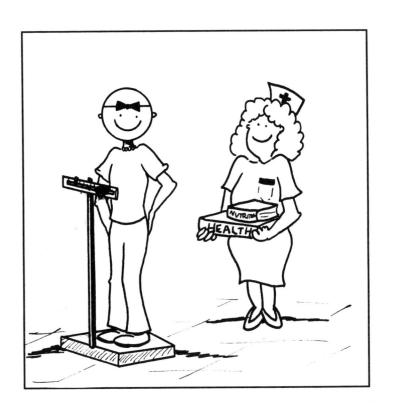

I have waited all my life for someone to tell me to eat!

A cancer diagnosis is not an automatic death sentence.

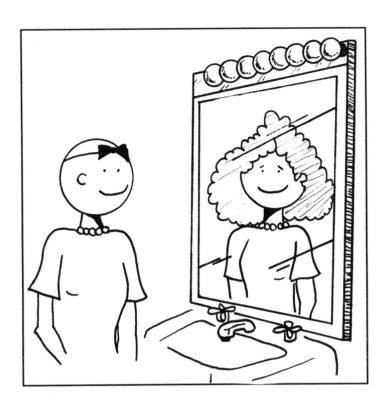

Gray hair wasn't so bad after all.

Anger. Talk about it and it will pass.

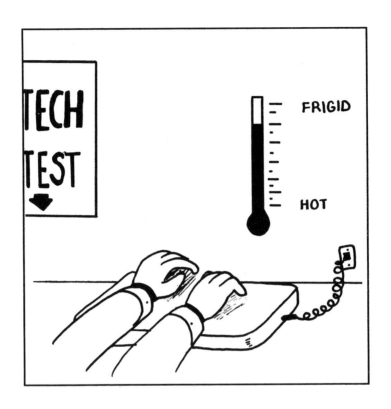

In order to be a tech you need to pass
the cold hands test.

Ask a question over and over until you feel comfortable with the answer.

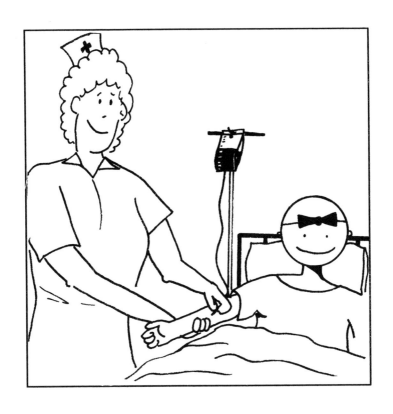

All I want for Christmas is another good vein.

Each day has at least one special moment. What was it today?

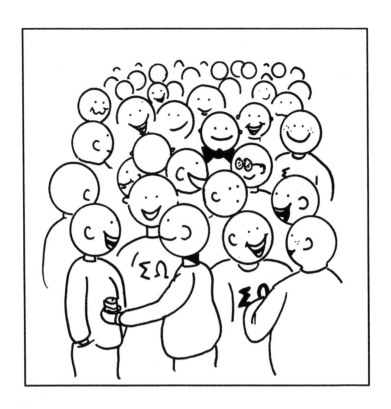

This is not the fraternity I dreamed
of joining.

It's nice to get a call asking what I'm doing rather than how I'm feeling. I'm not my disease.

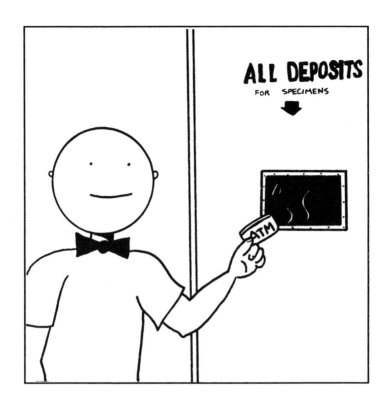

It says put all deposits here. I just never know where to put the ATM card.

I don't have to pay for this hospitalization.
I'm on the frequent bed program.

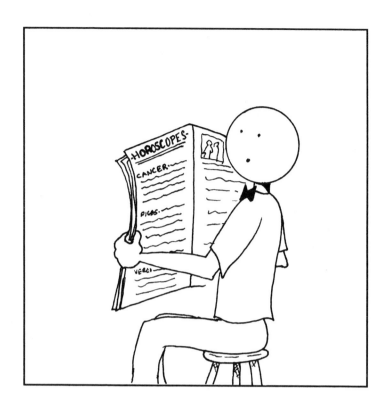

How can cancer be a disease if it's an astrological sign?

A hug says what words can't express.

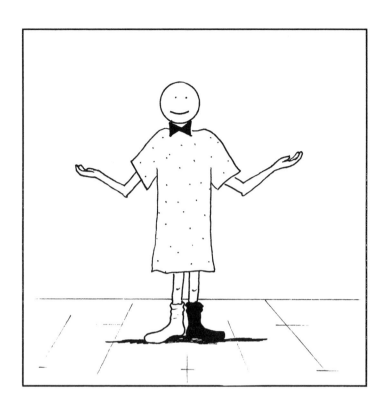

I can never remember if it's black or white socks that are appropriate for this type of outfit.

A teddy bear is blind to both gender and age.

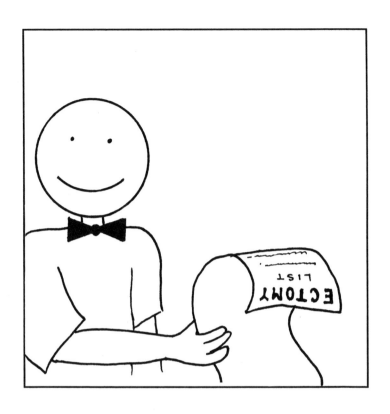

Some may call it a medical history.
I call it my *"ectomy"* list.

Only an octopus has enough hands to milk drains and measure fluids at the same time.

CHEMOTHERAPY GIVES NEW MEANING TO A BAD HAIR DAY

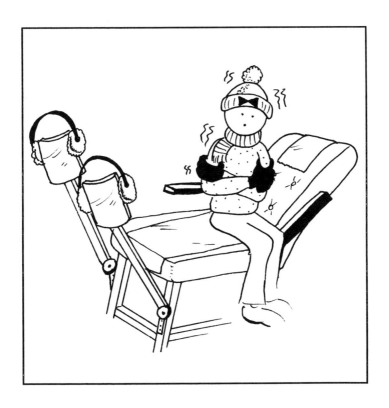

It's nice to have a compassionate doctor. Someone who cares if the stirrups are cold!

Use the pages that follow to
record your personal thoughts,
feelings and experiences.

Date the page and write a single
word, a sentence or scribble how
you feel or what's happened.

The pages are all yours.

Remember – there are no right or
wrong ways to be yourself –
on these pages or anywhere else!

Date _____

Date _____

Date _____

Date _____

Date _____

Date _____

Date _____

Date _____

*Date*_____

Date _____

Date _____

CHEMOTHERAPY GIVES NEW MEANING TO A BAD HAIR DAY

Date _____

Date _____

Date _____

Date _____

Date _____

Date _____

Date _____

Date _____

Date _____

Date _____